Sabaa Hilal Hadi
Mohamed Abdel-Raheem
Muna A. AL-Khafaji

Comparative Pathobiology of Viral Diseases in Farm Animals

Sabaa Hilal Hadi
Mohamed Abdel-Raheem
Muna A. AL-Khafaji

Comparative Pathobiology of Viral Diseases in Farm Animals

Second edition

Noor Publishing

Imprint

Cover image: www.ingimage.com

Publisher:
Noor Publishing
is a trademark of
Dodo Books Indian Ocean Ltd. and OmniScriptum S.R.L publishing group

120 High Road, East Finchley, London, N2 9ED, United Kingdom
Str. Armeneasca 28/1, office 1, Chisinau MD-2012, Republic of Moldova, Europe
Managing Directors: Ieva Konstantinova, Victoria Ursu
info@omniscriptum.com

Printed at: see last page
ISBN: 978-620-9-15325-9

Comparative Pathobiology of Viral Diseases in Farm Animals

Histopathological and Experimental Insights

Prof. Sabaa Hilal Hadi

Prof. Mohamed Abdel-Raheem

Prof. Dr. Muna. A. AL-Khafaji

Second Edition

2025

ORCID: https://orcid.org/0000-0003-2638-9408

Comparative Pathobiology of Viral Diseases in Farm Animals

Histopathological and Experimental Insights

By

Prof. Sabaa Hilal Hadi

Department of Pathology and Poultry Diseases

Faculty of Veterinary Medicine

Prof. Dr. Mohamed Abdel-Raheem Ali Abdel-Raheem

Professor of Biological Control

Pests & Plant Protection Department

Agricultural and Biological Research Institute

National Research Centre, Cairo, Egypt.

Prof. Dr. M.A. AL-KHAFAJI

Department of Pathology and Poultry Diseases, College of Veterinary Medicine, Al-Qasim Green University, Babylon 51013, Iraq.

muna200@vet.uoqasim.edu.iq

orcid.org/0000-0003-0022-0989

Second Edition

2025

First published in 2025 by

ISBN:

Printed in

This book is primarily based on a **peer-** published studies titled "Measurement of Iraqi
reviewed Infectious Dose for Aftosa Virus Sheep.", "Histological Changes in And
Isolated from Mice (Balb/c) Induced by "Histopathological and Hormonal
Newcastle Virus." Assessment of Contagious
Ecthyma in Rams."

The opinions expressed in this book are solely those of the author and do not necessarily reflect the views of any institution or organization.

About the Authors

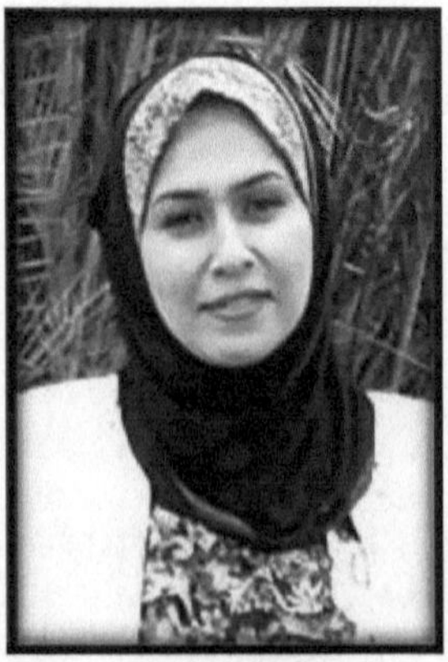

Prof. Sabaa Hilal Hadi

Department of Pathology and Poultry Diseases, Faculty of Veterinary Medicine, University of Al-Qasim Green, Babylon 51013, Iraq.

E-mail: sabahelal@vet.uoqasim.edu.iq

Professor **Sabaa Hilal Hadi** is a distinguished scholar whose expertise aligns closely with the scientific framework of this book. His extensive research in **microbiology, zoonotic diseases and veterinary pathology,** has contributed profoundly to understanding the mechanisms of host–pathogen interactions in animals. Through more than **27 peer-reviewed publications**, Professor Hadi has explored the pathological and microbiological aspects of major zoonotic agents such as *Enterobacter* and *Salmonella*, emphasizing their diagnostic, comparative, and public health implications. His academic endeavors complement the themes of **comparative pathobiology and**

experimental virology presented in this volume, enriching the broader discourse in veterinary biomedical research

Dedication

Dedicated to all veterinarians and researchers striving to improve animal heal

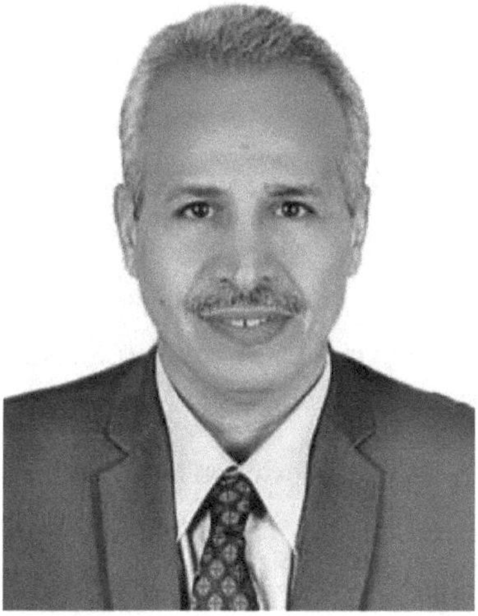

Prof. Dr. Mohamed Abdel-Raheem Ali Abdel-Raheem
Professor of Biological Control
Pests & Plant Protection Department
Agricultural and Biological Research Institute
National Research Centre.
33rd ElBohouth St., Dokki, Cairo, Egypt.
Email: abdelraheem_nrc@hotmail.com,
abdelraheem_nrc@yahoo.com

Prof. Dr. Mohamed Abdel-Raheem Ali Abdel-Raheem, Prof. of Entomology (Biological Control), Pests & Plant Protection Department, Agricultural and Biological Research Institute, National Research Centre, Cairo, Egypt. Published publications (316) papers (86), Books and Book chapters (229), Edited books (8), (Scopus) h-index (11), Citations (331), (Google Scholar) h-index (19) , Citations (1142), (Web of Science) Publications (28), h-index (11), Citations (295),

Research Gate, h-index (15), Citations (697), Reviewers in International Journals (156), Reviewed articles in Biological Control (1025), Editor in Chief in Journal (7), Assistant Editor (1), Associated Editor in Chief in Journal (7), Editorial board in Journals (42), Advisory board (1), conference Attended (27), workshop Attended (308), Symposium Attended (179), Forum Attended (4), Prize (4), Attended Others (30), Projects As PI and member (20), Training courses For Agric. Engineering (61), Training courses For Students of University (8), attending Trainees courses (19), TV, Radio & Newspaper (35), Supervisor on Ms.C. thesis (3), Supervisor on Ph.D. thesis (1), Committee Ph.D. Thesis in Egypt (2), and member in scientific Foundation (14), Giving International lectures (4), Promotion Committee Prof. international (1), Committee Ph.D. thesis international (1).

National Research Centre. 33rd ElBohouth St., Dokki, Cairo, Egypt.

Email Address: abdelraheem_nrc@hotmail.com, ma.abdel-raheem@nrc.sci.eg, abdelraheem_nrc@yahoo.com, profmohamedabdelraheem@gmail.com, abdelraheem196942@gmail.com, mabdelraheem69@gmail.com, mabdelraheem69@yahoo.com.

Mobile Phone: (+2) 01155527583 – (+2) 01009580797

Scopus Author ID : 55220661700

https://www.scopus.com/authid/detail.uri?authorId=55220661700

http://scholar.google.com/citations?hl=en&user=gBtssEgAAAAJ

https://orcid.org/my-orcid?orcid=0000-0001-9240-064X

https://www.webofscience.com/wos/author/searchAbdel-Raheem, Mohamed Abdel-Raheem Ali - Web of Science Core Collection

https://www.researchgate.net/profile/Mohamed_Abdel-Raheem4/publications?sorting=recentlyAdded

http://livedna.org/20.16018

http://www.resarcherid.com/rid/R-6264-2017

https://www.webofscience.com/wos/author/record/R-6264-2017

https://www.facebook.com/share/p/1Piu6xyFmN/

- TV, Radio & Newspaper links

1. https://www.youtube.com/attribution_link?a=NsH2xGv9mY8&u=%2Fwatch%3Fv%3Dsb46rBG8-Mc%26feature%3Dshare
2. https://youtu.be/Ub8djW0tggo
3. https://m.facebook.com/story.php?story_fbid=492907069288338&id=100076011247165
4. https://youtu.be/dOujUAZmTdw
5. https://m.facebook.com/story.php?story_fbid=492907069288338&id=100076011247165
6. https://fb.watch/gPGrDuzZFX/
7. https://www.youtube.com/watch?si=4UfyQaeHVLPiVR5J&v=nXV4NT-no7o&feature=youtu.be
8. https://www.youtube.com/watch?v=sRH44W6TbcQ
9. https://youtu.be/uq9Qj3AEBHk?si=ymaX06huG2AXJESu
10. https://www.facebook.com/share/v/Qg5s6HW3hD8PLBzp/?mibextid=xfxF2i
11. https://el-yom.com/news/archives/1092767
12. https://el-yomnews.com/?p=1156515
13. https://el-yomnews.com/%D8%A7%D9%84%D8%AF%D9%83%D8%AA%D9%88%D8%B1-%D8%B9%D8%A8%D8%AF%D8%A7%D9%84%D8%B1%D8%AD%D9%8A%D9%85-%D9%85%D8%AD%D9%85%D8%AF-%D8%B9%D9%84%D9%8A-

%D9%8A%D8%AA%D8%AD%D8%AF%D8%AB-%D9%84-%D9%84%D9%84/

14. https://el-yomnews.com/?p=1179515
15. https://www.facebook.com/share/v/4MM85wKRPxsYLqTr/
16. http://https//el-yomnews.com/%D8%A7%D9%84%D8%AD%D8%B4%D8%B1%D8%A7%D8%AA-%D9%81%D9%8A-%D8%AE%D8%AF%D9%85%D8%A9-%D8%A7%D9%84%D8%B9%D8%AF%D8%A7%D9%84%D8%A9-%D9%85%D8%AD%D8%A7%D8%B6%D8%B1%D8%A9-%D8%AA%D9%83%D8%B4%D9%81-%D8%AF%D9%88/
17. https://youtube.com/watch?v=F21ziQxdeco&si=LvSUixmnSg4JM1zK
18. https://youtu.be/F21ziQxdeco?si=jyAwbU8dVwkYzRH4

19- https://el-yomnews.com/المكافحة-الحيوية-بالفطريات-حلول-مبتك/

20- https://el-yomnews.com/archives/1296404

21- https://www.facebook.com/share/p/1AC25ue5XG/

22- https://youtu.be/7VItE5kON2g?si=9rMWMUSGk8Csgjfn

23- https://www.youtube.com/watch?v=G9nXA7Q9C60

24- https://www.youtube.com/watch?v=7VItE5kON2g

25- https://el-yomnews.com/archives/1347977

26- https://youtu.be/x9N58DakONg?si=Uh0HbpQsiDRpIGMl

27- https://youtu.be/PfuQy-Zkq3s?si=GtRRxy9XtTW-YgF3

TV and Radio

1- Filming in the program (Meeting the Scientists) - Al-Manara Channel, entitled Biological Control of Insect Pests, on 7/2/2013.

2- Filming in the program (Friends of Al-Manara) - Al-Manara Channel, February 2014.

3- A recording of an interview with the program (From the Secrets of the Universe and Life) Radio Sawt Al-Arab, Cairo on 4/26/2015.

4- Filming in the program (Idea for a bobbin) - Nile Cultural Channel under the title "Using entomopathogenic fungi and plant extracts in combating insect pests that infect sugar crops in Egypt" on 11/1/2015.

5- Filming on (This Morning) program - Nile News Channel under the title: Submitting the specifications for the reclamation of one and a half million feddans as a first stage of the reclamation of 4 million feddans on 11/15/2015. https://www.youtube.com/attribution_link?a=NsH2xGv9mY8&u=%2Fwatch%3Fv%3Dsb46rBG8-Mc%26feature%3Dshare

6- Registration in the program (Our Life Between Our Hands) for North Upper Egypt Radio and Radio, presented by Dr. Essam Fathy, 3 episodes, on 11-29-2021, and it will be broadcast on Saturday and Wednesday at 3:30 pm in January 2022

7- Registration in the program (Our Life Between Our Hands) for North Upper Egypt Radio and Radio, presented by Dr. Essam Fathy, 3 episodes, on 11-29-2021, and it will be broadcast on Saturday and Wednesday at 3:30 pm in January 2022

8- Registration in the program (Our Life Between Our Hands) for North Upper Egypt Radio and Radio, presented by Dr. Essam Fathy, 3 episodes, on 11-29-2021, and it will be broadcast on Saturday and Wednesday at 3:30 pm in January 2022

9- Registration in "Our Green Land" program for North Upper Egypt Radio and Radio, presented by Dr. Essam Fathy, 3 episodes, on 11-2021-2021, to be broadcast in January 2022

10- Registration in "Our Green Land" program for North Upper Egypt Radio and Radio, presented by Dr. Essam Fathy, 3 episodes, on 11-2021-2021, to be broadcast in January 2022
11- Registration in "Our Green Land" program for North Upper Egypt Radio and Radio, presented by Dr. Essam Fathy, 3 episodes, on 11-2021-2021, to be broadcast in January 2022
12- Filming in the program (Egypt is Beautiful) - the second Egyptian Nile Channel, under the title: Climate Changes on November 6, 2022. https://youtu.be/dOujUAZmTdw
13- Registration in "Our Green Land" program for North Upper Egypt Radio and Radio, presented by Dr. Essam Fathy, 3 episodes, on 11-2021-2021, to be broadcast in January 2022
14- Filming in the program (Egypt and Climate Summit) - Delta Satellite Channel under the title: Climate Cop 27 on 13/11/2022 https://youtu.be/Ub8djW0tggo
15- Filming in (Egypt) - Sohag, Coral Times Hotel, under the title: Climate Change, Cop 27, dated 11/15/2022, the journalist Shorouk Abdullah https://m.facebook.com/story.php?story_fbid=492907069288338&id=100076011247165
16- Filming in (Feed and Benefit) - Coral Hotel in Sohag under the title: Climate Cop 27 on 11/15/2022, journalist Ahmed Tarboush https://fb.watch/gPGrDuzZFX/
17- An intervention in the plant clinic program on insect-pathogenic fungi in Egypt's agricultural farms on Thursday 29/2/2024. https://www.youtube.com/watch?si=4UfyQaeHVLPiVR5J&v=nXV4NT-no7o&feature=youtu.be
18- Filming in the plant clinic program on the Misr Agricultural Channel about insect-pathogenic fungi on Sunday 3-3-2024

https://www.youtube.com/watch?v=sRH44W6TbcQ

19- Filming in the plant clinic program at the Misr Agricultural Channel, early prediction of the red palm weevil and modern methods of combating it, on Thursday 25/4/2024.
https://youtu.be/uq9Qj3AEBHk?si=ymaX06huG2AXJESu

20- Filming in the Green Planet program on the Egyptian Channel 2 (Biological Control) on Sunday 7/6/2024
https://www.facebook.com/watch/?v=981454710052376

21- A press interview in Al-Youm newspaper with journalist Mr. Imad Naseer on 7-30-2024. https://el-yom.com/news/archives/1092767
https://el-yomnews.com/

22- https://el-yomnews.com/?p=1156515

23- https://el-yomnews.com/%D8%A7%D9%84%D8%AF%D9%83%D8%AA%D9%88%D8%B1-%D8%B9%D8%A8%D8%AF%D8%A7%D9%84%D8%B1%D8%AD%D9%8A%D9%85-%D9%85%D8%AD%D9%85%D8%AF-%D8%B9%D9%84%D9%8A-%D9%8A%D8%AA%D8%AD%D8%AF%D8%AB-%D9%84-%D9%84%D9%84/

24- https://el-yomnews.com/?p=1179515

25- https://www.facebook.com/share/v/4MM85wKRPxsYLqTr/

26- Insects in the Service of Justice: A Lecture Explaining the Role of Forensic Entomology in Investigating Crimes
https://el-yomnews.com/archives/1243894

27- Human health is at risk. An investigation reveals the secrets of pesticide-contaminated agriculture.

https://el-yomnews.com/archives/1296404

28- https://www.facebook.com/share/p/1AC25ue5XG/

The Green Planet Program (Beneficial Insects and Their Role in the Environment) on 5/23/2025 on the Egyptian Channel 2

29- https://youtu.be/7VItE5kON2g?si=9rMWMUSGk8Csgjfn

30- https://www.youtube.com/watch?v=G9nXA7Q9C60

31- https://www.youtube.com/watch?v=7VItE5kON2g

32- https://el-yomnews.com/archives/1347977

33- https://youtu.be/x9N58DakONg?si=Uh0HbpQsiDRpIGMl

https://youtu.be/PfuQy-Zkq3s?si=GtRRxy9XtTW-YgF3

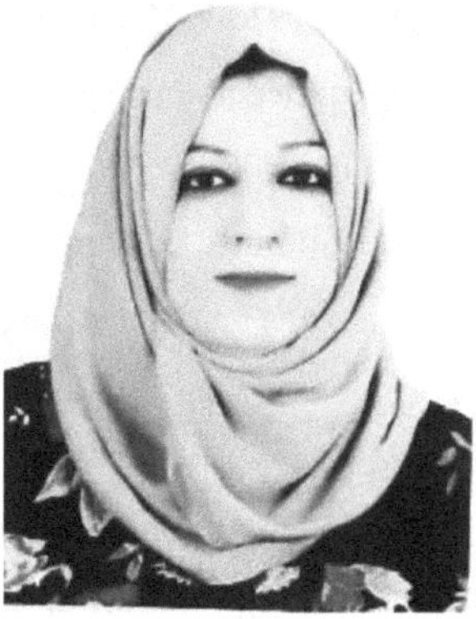

Muna. A. AL-Khafaji , ***DVM, PhD***
Professor of Pathology
Department of Pathology and Poultry Diseases, College of Veterinary Medicine, Al-Qasim Green University, Babylon 51013, Iraq.
E- mail: muna200@vet.uoqasim.edu.iq

Preface

The field of veterinary virology continues to evolve rapidly as emerging pathogens challenge global food security and animal welfare. This book, *Comparative Pathobiology of Viral Diseases in Farm Animals*, was developed to bridge the gap between experimental research and practical applications in veterinary pathology. It integrates histopathological, hormonal, and immunological findings from multiple viral systems, offering a comparative view that enhances understanding of cross-species disease dynamics.

The chapters within this volume are structured to guide readers from general concepts to specific case studies, culminating in a comparative synthesis of major viral pathogens— Foot-and-Mouth Disease Virus (FMDV), Newcastle Disease Virus (NDV), and Orf Virus (ORFV). Each chapter draws from peer-reviewed research and experimental data, with an emphasis on clarity, accessibility, and scientific rigor.

The authors hopes that this book will serve as a valuable reference for veterinary students, researchers, and professionals seeking a deeper understanding of animal viral pathology and its translational implications for public and animal health.

Prof. Sabaa Hilal Hadi
Prof. Mohamed Abdel-Raheem
Prof. Dr. M.A. AL-KHAFAJI

Table of Contents

Chapter 1 – General Introduction to Animal Viral Pathology - Comparative Pathobiology of Viral Diseases

Chapter 1 – General Introduction to Animal Viral Pathology

Book Overview

This chapter provides an introductory framework for understanding animal viral pathology with emphasis on the comparative aspects of Foot-and-Mouth Disease Virus (FMDV), Newcastle Disease Virus (NDV), and Contagious Ecthyma Virus (ORFV). It integrates epidemiological, immunological, and experimental perspectives to form the foundation for subsequent chapters that examine each virus in detail.

1.1 Introduction to Veterinary Virology

Veterinary virology is a cornerstone discipline within veterinary medicine and animal health sciences. It investigates the biology, transmission, and pathogenesis of viruses affecting livestock and wildlife populations. Animal viruses can cause devastating economic and social impacts, especially in developing countries where agriculture and animal husbandry are major livelihood sources (Sumption et al., 2008). Understanding the nature of these pathogens is critical to designing effective control strategies and preventive vaccination programs.

1.2 Economic and Health Importance of Animal Viral Diseases

The global livestock industry experiences billions of dollars in annual losses due to viral diseases. Foot-and-mouth disease (FMD), for instance, remains among the most economically important transboundary animal diseases (Beure, 2013). Newcastle disease significantly reduces poultry productivity and trade potential (Alexander, 2003), while contagious ecthyma affects small ruminant health and poses zoonotic threats to humans (Nandi et al., 2011). In addition to direct mortality, viral outbreaks result in decreased fertility, reduced milk and meat yield, and high costs of vaccination and quarantine.

1.3 Concept of Comparative Pathobiology

Comparative pathobiology focuses on identifying similarities and differences in disease processes among various species and viruses. Through histopathological and molecular comparisons, researchers can reveal shared mechanisms of tissue damage and host responses. In this book, the comparative analysis of FMDV, NDV, and ORFV highlights how diverse viruses employ similar strategies of infection, replication, and immune evasion within different host systems.

1.4 Overview of the Studied Viruses (FMDV, NDV, ORFV)

Foot-and-Mouth Disease Virus (FMDV) is a member of the Picornaviridae family, genus Aphthovirus, characterized by a positive-sense RNA genome. It infects cloven-hoofed animals such as cattle, sheep, and goats. Newcastle Disease Virus (NDV), belonging to Paramyxoviridae, is an avian pathogen with zoonotic potential, known to cause respiratory and neurological manifestations in birds and mild conjunctivitis in humans (Alexander, 2003). Contagious ecthyma (Orf) virus is a Parapoxvirus that causes proliferative skin lesions in sheep and goats, occasionally transmitted to humans (Nandi et al., 2011).

Figure 1. Comparative morphology and genomic structure of FMDV, NDV, and ORFV

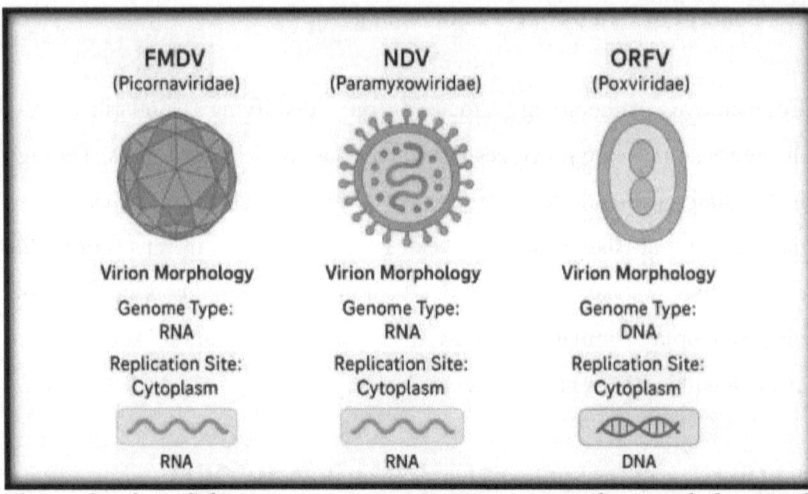

Figure Caption: *Schematic representation comparing the morphology and genomic architecture of three major farm animal viruses: Foot-and-Mouth Disease Virus (FMDV), Newcastle Disease Virus (NDV), and Orf Virus (ORFV). FMDV (Picornaviridae) is a small, non-enveloped icosahedral RNA virus; NDV (Paramyxoviridae) is an enveloped pleomorphic RNA virus with surface glycoproteins; and ORFV (Poxviridae) is a large, enveloped DNA virus with complex lateral bodies. The figure highlights differences in genome type, replication site, and virion morphology.*

1.5 Mechanisms of Viral Pathogenesis in Animals

The mechanisms of viral pathogenesis involve a complex interplay between viral virulence factors and host immune defenses. Following infection, viruses attach to host cell receptors, penetrate membranes, and exploit cellular machinery to replicate. Histopathological changes such as necrosis, cellular degeneration, and vascular congestion are common outcomes of infection (Thayer & Beard, 2008). The studied viruses display distinct tropisms—FMDV targets epithelial tissues, NDV targets the gastrointestinal and respiratory tracts, while ORFV primarily affects the skin and reproductive organs.

Chapter 1 – General Introduction to Animal Viral Pathology - Comparative Pathobiology of Viral Diseases

1.6 Advances in Experimental and Diagnostic Techniques

Modern veterinary virology employs a variety of diagnostic tools such as polymerase chain

reaction (PCR), enzyme-linked immunosorbent assay (ELISA), and immunohistochemistry (IHC). In experimental pathology, embryonated chicken eggs, laboratory mice, and farm animals are utilized as model systems to assess viral infectivity and tissue responses (Reed & Muench, 1938). The integration of histopathological and molecular techniques improves diagnostic accuracy and aids in vaccine development.

Table 1. Summary of diagnostic and experimental techniques used in veterinary virology

Technique	Principle	Common Application	Example Virus
Virus Isolation	Growth in embryonated eggs or cell cultures to detect cytopathic effect (CPE).	Confirming infectivity and strain identification.	FMDV, NDV
Histopathology	Tissue sectioning and staining (H&E, special stains) to visualize lesions.	Routine diagnosis and pathological grading.	NDV, ORFV
Serological Tests (ELISA, VNT)	Detection of viral antigens or antibodies.	Epidemiological surveys and vaccine response.	FMDV
Molecular Techniques (PCR, RT-PCR, qPCR)	Amplification and quantification of viral	Rapid diagnosis and genotyping.	FMDV, NDV

	nucleic acids.		
Immunohistochemistry (IHC)	Antibody-based labeling of viral proteins in tissues.	Localization of virus within lesions.	ORFV
Electron Microscopy	Visualization of virion morphology.	Confirmation of novel or atypical viruses.	FMDV, ORFV
Next-Generation Sequencing (NGS)	High-throughput genome analysis.	Molecular epidemiology and strain evolution.	FMDV, NDV, ORFV

Table Caption: Summary of key laboratory techniques employed in the diagnosis and research of major viral diseases in farm animals. Each technique contributes unique diagnostic information—ranging from morphological to molecular—supporting integrated approaches in veterinary virology.

1.7 Immune Responses to Viral Infections

Host immunity against viral pathogens involves both innate and adaptive components. Innate immunity acts as the first line of defense through interferons, macrophages, and natural killer cells. Adaptive immunity, mediated by T and B lymphocytes, provides antigen-specific responses and immunological memory. The balance between these systems determines disease outcome. For instance, NDV induces both mucosal and systemic immunity in birds, whereas ORFV modulates local immune responses to persist within epithelial tissues (Bennett et al., 2016).

1.8 Challenges and Future Perspectives in Veterinary Virology

Despite advances in molecular diagnostics and vaccine production, challenges persist in eradicating viral diseases from livestock. Viral mutation rates, antigenic diversity, and environmental persistence complicate control programs. Additionally, limited biosecurity and poor veterinary infrastructure in certain regions hinder outbreak management. Future research should emphasize cross-species studies, genomic surveillance, and the development of broad-spectrum antiviral agents (Akhigbe et al., 2022).

Chapter Summary

This introductory chapter establishes a foundation for understanding the comparative pathology of animal viral diseases. By exploring the biology, pathogenesis, and immune responses associated with FMDV, NDV, and ORFV, the reader gains a conceptual framework for interpreting the experimental and histopathological findings detailed in the following chapters.

List of Figures and Tables

References

Alexander, D. J. (2003). Newcastle disease and other avian paramyxoviruses. Rev. Sci.

Tech. Off. Int. Epiz., 19(2), 443–462.

Akhigbe, R. E., Dutta, S., Hamed, M. A., Ajayi, A. F., Sengupta, P., & Ahmad, G. (2022). Viral infections and male infertility: A comprehensive review of oxidative stress. Frontiers in Reproductive Health, 4, 782915.

Beure, K. (2013). Canadian Food Inspection Agency report on foot and mouth disease transmission and control. CFIA Publications.

Bennett, J. R., Lateef, Z., Fleming, S. B., Mercer, A. A., & Wise, L. M. (2016). Orf virus IL-10 reduces monocyte, dendritic cell, and mast cell recruitment to inflamed skin. Virus Research, 213, 230–237.

Nandi, S., De, U. K., & Chowdhury, S. (2011). Current status of contagious ecthyma (orf disease) in goats and sheep: A global perspective. Small Ruminant Research, 96(2), 73– 82.

Chapter 1 – General Introduction to Animal Viral Pathology - Comparative Pathobiology of Viral Diseases

Reed, L. J., & Muench, H. (1938). A simple method of estimating fifty percent endpoints.

American Journal of Hygiene, 27, 493–497.

Sumption, K., Rweyemamu, M., & Wint, W. (2008). Incidence and distribution of foot-and-mouth disease in Asia, Africa, and South America. Transboundary and Emerging Diseases, 55(1), 5–13.

Thayer, S. G., & Beard, C. W. (2008). Serologic procedures. In A Laboratory Manual for the Identification and Characterization of Avian Pathogens (5th ed., pp. 222–229). American Association of Avian Pathologists.

Chapter 2 – Methodological Approaches in Veterinary Virology - Comparative Pathobiology of Viral Diseases

Chapter 2 – Methodological Approaches in Veterinary Virology

2.1 Overview

This chapter discusses the experimental and diagnostic methodologies employed in veterinary virology. It outlines the principles behind sample collection, virus isolation, animal experimentation, histopathological preparation, and molecular techniques that form the basis of comparative viral pathology. These methods are essential for understanding the infectivity, tissue tropism, and pathogenic behavior of viruses such as FMDV, NDV, and ORFV.

2.2 Sample Collection and Handling

The foundation of successful virological studies depends heavily on appropriate sample collection and preservation. Samples must represent the stage and site of infection accurately. For FMDV, epithelial tissue and vesicular fluid from lesions are preferred; for NDV, fecal material, tracheal swabs, and organ tissues are suitable; for ORFV, scab materials and lesion biopsies are standard specimens (Sumption et al., 2008; Nandi et al., 2011). Samples should be transported in viral transport medium at 4°C and processed promptly to preserve viral viability.

2.3 Virus Isolation and Propagation

Virus isolation remains the gold standard for confirming active infection. Embryonated chicken eggs (9–11 days old) are used extensively for FMDV and NDV propagation. The chorioallantoic membrane (CAM) and allantoic cavity routes are selected depending on the virus type (Alexander, 2003). For ORFV, primary cell cultures such as lamb testis or bovine kidney cells are ideal for viral growth (Beure, 2013). Each inoculation is performed under sterile conditions, and embryos or cultures are incubated at 37°C for 3–7 days, followed by harvesting of viral suspensions.

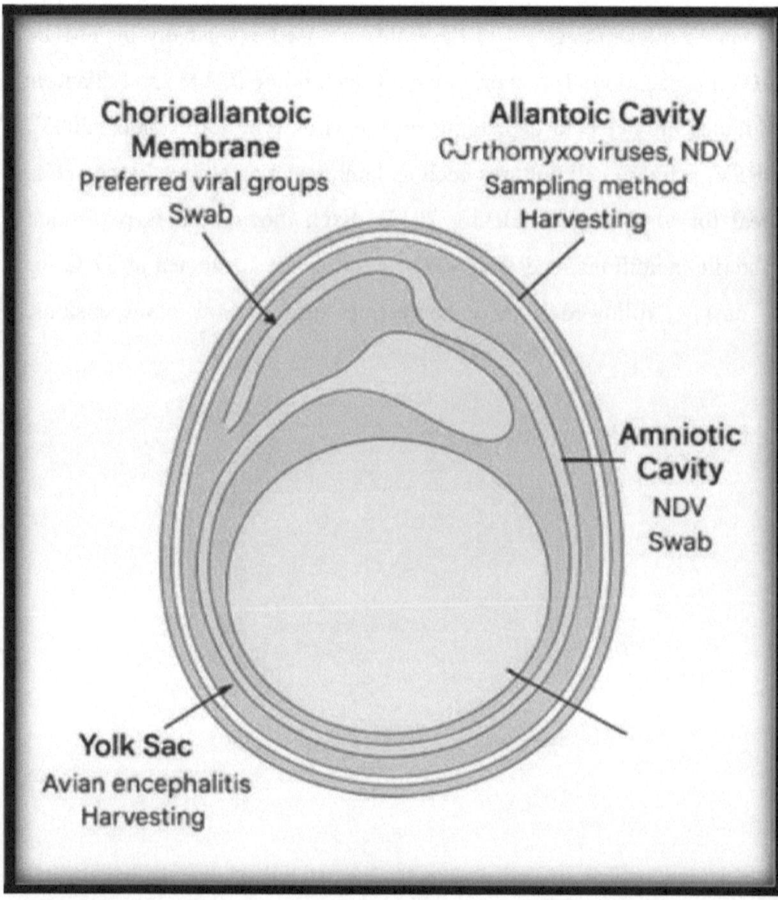

Figure 2. Overview of inoculation routes in embryonated chicken eggs

Figure caption: *Illustration depicting the main inoculation routes used in embryonated chicken eggs for viral propagation: chorioallantoic membrane (CAM), allantoic cavity, amniotic cavity, and yolk sac. Each route is labeled with its preferred viral groups and sampling method. The diagram highlights how route selection influences viral yield and tissue tropism.*

2.4 Animal Experimentation Models

Animal models are indispensable in veterinary virology for studying pathogenicity and immune response. Laboratory mice, sheep, and poultry species serve as experimental hosts. Mice (Balb/c) are used to evaluate tissue reactions to NDV, while embryonated eggs are employed to determine the infectious dose of FMDV (Reed & Muench, 1938). Ethical considerations are paramount, and all procedures must adhere to international animal welfare standards and institutional biosafety protocols.

Table 2. Commonly used animal models and their applications in viral pathogenesis studies

Animal Model	**Representative**	**Research**		**Advantages**
	Virus	**Applicati on**		
Embryonated	FMDV, NDV	Virus	isolation ,	Easy to handle,
Chicken Egg		titration		reproducible results
Mouse (Balb/c)	NDV	Pathogenesis,		Well-characterized
		histology		immune system

Sheep/Rams	ORFV	Natural host infection models	Reflects real field conditions
Guinea Pig	FMDV	Immune response evaluation	Suitable for vaccine testing
Cell Culture (Vero, BHK-21)	FMDV, NDV	In vitro and cytopathology	Controlled environment

Table caption: *Summary of animal models commonly employed in experimental virology. Each model offers unique advantages for studying host–pathogen interactions and disease progression.*

2.5 Histopathological Examination and Tissue Processing

Histopathological analysis provides direct evidence of tissue damage and cellular alterations caused by viral infection. Tissues are fixed in 10% neutral buffered formalin for 24–48 hours, dehydrated in graded alcohols, embedded in paraffin, and sectioned at 4–6 μm thickness. Slides are stained using hematoxylin and eosin (H&E) and examined microscopically. Special stains such as immunohistochemical labeling may be employed to detect viral antigens (Thayer & Beard, 2008).

Figure 3. Workflow of tissue fixation and staining in veterinary pathology

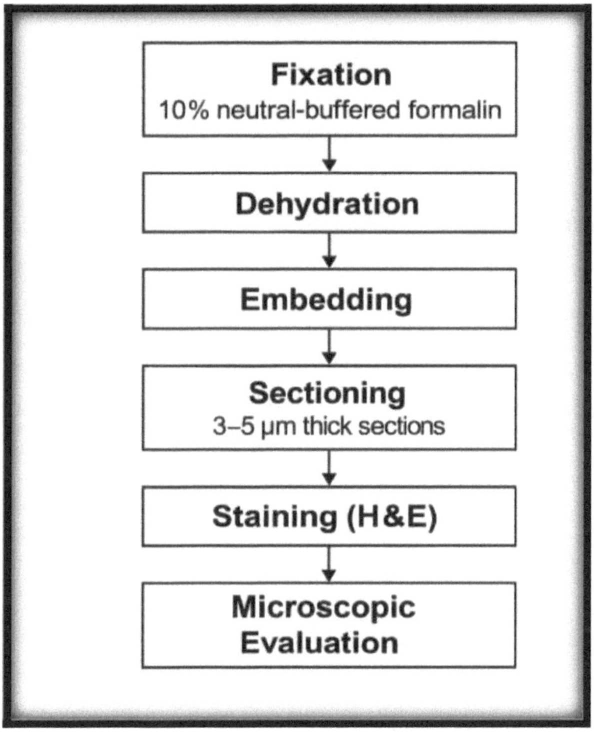

Figure caption: Flow diagram outlining the sequential steps in tissue processing for histopathological examination: fixation, dehydration, embedding, sectioning, staining (H&E), and microscopic evaluation.

The figure also indicates critical parameters such as fixative concentration and section thickness.

Chapter 2 – Methodological Approaches in Veterinary Virology - Comparative Pathobiology of Viral Diseases

2.6 Molecular and Immunological Techniques

Molecular diagnostics have revolutionized viral detection and characterization. Techniques such as polymerase chain reaction (PCR), quantitative PCR (qPCR), and sequencing allow rapid identification of viral genomes. Serological tests like ELISA and virus neutralization assays are used to quantify antibody responses. In the case of ORFV, PCR targeting the ORFV037 gene provides specific confirmation of infection (Nandi et al., 2011). The integration of molecular and immunological methods enhances both sensitivity and specificity of diagnostics.

2.7 Data Analysis and Statistical Evaluation

Quantitative analysis of experimental data, including viral titers, lesion scores, and histological indices, requires statistical rigor. The Reed and Muench (1938) method is used to calculate the 50% Embryo Infectious Dose (EID50), while ANOVA and t-tests are applied for comparing group differences. Data visualization through graphs and histograms aids interpretation and enhances clarity of presentation.

Figure 4. Example of EID50 calculation curve for FMDV infection

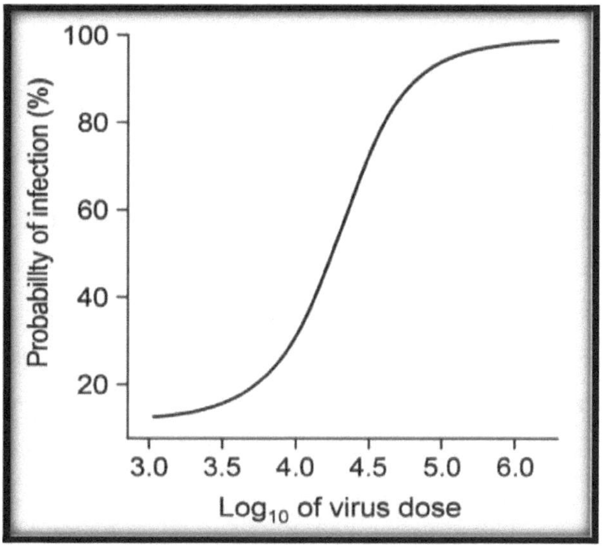

Figure caption: Graphical plot illustrating a typical 50% egg infectious dose (EID_{50}) calculation using the Reed–Muench method. The x-axis represents dilution factors (10^{-1} to 10^{-6}), while the y-axis represents percentage infection rate. The intersection point identifies the dilution corresponding to 50% infection probability.

Chapter 2 – Methodological Approaches in Veterinary Virology - Comparative Pathobiology of Viral Diseases

2.8 Biosafety and Ethical Considerations

Working with infectious agents requires strict adherence to biosafety levels (BSL) appropriate for each pathogen. FMDV and NDV typically require BSL-3 facilities, whereas ORFV may be handled in BSL-2 with appropriate personal protective equipment. Personnel should undergo biosafety training, and waste materials must be decontaminated via autoclaving or chemical disinfection. All experimental designs involving animals must be approved by an Institutional Animal Care and Use Committee (IACUC).

2.9 Emerging Technologies in Veterinary Virology

Recent innovations such as metagenomic sequencing, CRISPR-based diagnostics, and nanotechnology-assisted biosensors are transforming veterinary virology. These methods allow detection of unknown or emerging viral strains, monitor genomic evolution, and improve real-time surveillance (Akhigbe et al., 2022). Artificial intelligence (AI) and machine learning are also being employed to predict viral outbreaks and analyze histopathological images with higher precision.

Table 3. Comparison of conventional and emerging diagnostic technologies

Diagnostic Category	**Conventional Method**	**Emerging Method**	**Key Improvement**
Virus Detection	Egg inoculation	RT-qPCR, NGS	Rapid and sensitive detection
Serology	ELISA	Multiplex immunoassays	Higher throughput, specificity
Histopathology	H&E staining	Digital pathology with AI analysis	Quantitative lesion scoring
Viral Typing	Neutralization tests	Genomic sequencing	Strain-level identification
Field Diagnosis	Lateral flow tests	CRISPR-based biosensors	On-site precision diagnostics

Table caption: Comparison between traditional and modern diagnostic approaches in veterinary virology, emphasizing how molecular and digital tools are reshaping disease investigation.

Chapter Summary

This chapter summarized the principal methodologies applied in veterinary virology. From sample collection to molecular diagnostics, each technique contributes uniquely to the understanding of viral behavior and disease mechanisms. Integrating traditional pathological assessments with modern molecular technologies enhances diagnostic

Chapter 2 – Methodological Approaches in Veterinary Virology - Comparative Pathobiology of Viral Diseases

References

Alexander, D. J. (2003). Newcastle disease and other avian paramyxoviruses. Rev. Sci. Tech. Off. Int. Epiz., 19(2), 443–462.

Akhigbe, R. E., Dutta, S., Hamed, M. A., Ajayi, A. F., Sengupta, P., & Ahmad, G. (2022). Viral infections and male infertility: A comprehensive review of oxidative stress. Frontiers in Reproductive Health, 4, 782915.

Beure, K. (2013). Canadian Food Inspection Agency report on foot and mouth disease transmission and control. CFIA Publications.

Nandi, S., De, U. K., & Chowdhury, S. (2011). Current status of contagious ecthyma (orf disease) in goats and sheep: A global perspective. Small Ruminant Research, 96(2), 73– 82.

Reed, L. J., & Muench, H. (1938). A simple method of estimating fifty percent endpoints. American Journal of Hygiene, 27, 493–497.

Sumption, K., Rweyemamu, M., & Wint, W. (2008). Incidence and distribution of foot-and-mouth disease in Asia, Africa, and South America. Transboundary and Emerging Diseases, 55(1), 5–13.

Thayer, S. G., & Beard, C. W. (2008). Serologic procedures. In A Laboratory Manual for the Identification and Characterization of Avian Pathogens (5th ed., pp. 222–229). American Association of Avian Pathologists.

Chapter 3 – Experimental Assessment of Foot-and-Mouth Disease Virus (FMDV) - Comparative Pathobiology of Viral Diseases

Chapter 3 – Experimental Assessment of Foot-and-Mouth Disease Virus (FMDV)

Relation to Original Research

This chapter is primarily based on the peer review published study titled "Measurement of Infectious Dose for Aftosa Virus Isolated from Iraqi Sheep." The chapter expands on its experimental findings and integrates them with global literature on foot-and-mouth disease virus (FMDV) to provide a comparative and comprehensive interpretation of the infection process, embryonic model evaluation, and histopathological observations.

3.1 Background

Foot-and-Mouth Disease Virus (FMDV) is a highly contagious RNA virus that affects cloven-hoofed animals including cattle, sheep, goats, and pigs. It is classified under the genus Aphthovirus within the Picornaviridae family. FMDV causes vesicular lesions in the mouth, feet, and teats, leading to severe economic losses in livestock industries worldwide (Sumption et al., 2008). The disease's rapid spread and antigenic variability make it a constant threat in endemic regions.

3.2 Epidemiology and Significance

FMDV remains endemic in several regions of Asia, the Middle East, and Africa. Iraq has reported periodic outbreaks that affect small ruminant populations and threaten neighboring countries due to cross-border animal movement. Transmission occurs primarily through direct contact with infected secretions and aerosols, but mechanical transmission via vehicles, equipment, and humans also plays a role (Knight-Jones & Rushton, 2013). The virus's persistence in the environment complicates eradication efforts.

3.3 Experimental Design and Methods

The experiment followed standard embryonated chicken egg inoculation techniques to determine the 50% Embryo Infectious Dose (EID50). Fifty embryonated chicken eggs aged 9–11 days were divided equally into infected and control groups. The infected group received 0.2 mL of a FMDV suspension diluted in phosphate-buffered saline, while the control group received only the buffer solution. All eggs were incubated at 37°C and observed for up to 72 hours post-inoculation for mortality and embryonic lesions.

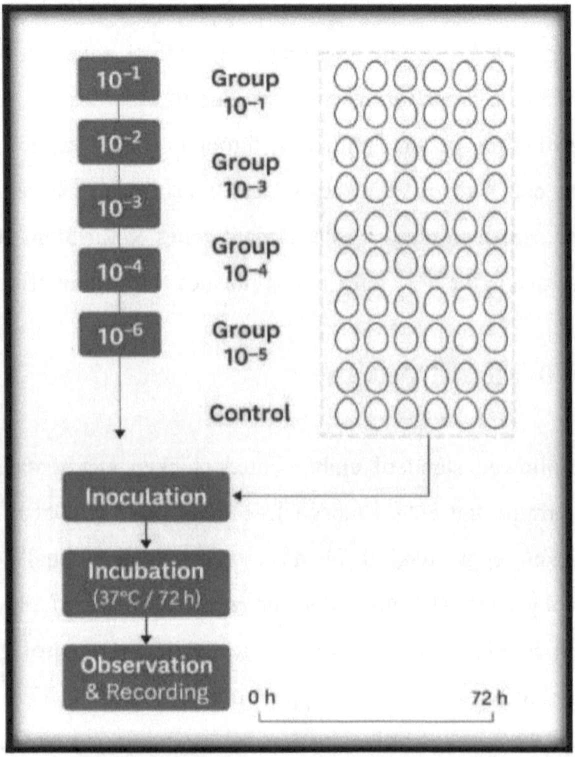

Figure 5. Experimental design for FMDV inoculation in embryonated chicken eggs

Figure caption: Diagram illustrating the experimental layout for determining the infectious dose (EID_{50}) of Foot-and-Mouth Disease Virus (FMDV) using embryonated chicken eggs. The figure shows division of eggs into groups based on dilution series (10^{-1} to 10^{-6}), inoculation routes, incubation period (37°C for 72 h), and subsequent mortality observation. Control eggs receive sterile buffer only.

3.4 Determination of EID_{50}

The infectivity titer of FMDV was determined using the Reed and Muench (1938) method to calculate the 50% Embryo Infectious Dose (EID50). Serial tenfold dilutions of the viral suspension were prepared, and mortality data from the inoculated embryos were used to compute EID50 values. The calculated titer was $10^{4.7}$ EID50/mL, indicating high viral infectivity. This level of infectivity aligns with previously reported titers for Asian serotypes of FMDV (Paton et al., 2009).

Table 4. EID_{50} calculation for FMDV using serial dilutions

Dilution (10^{-x})	**No. of Eggs Inoculated**	**No. of Infected Embryos**	**% Infection**	**Cumulative % Mortality**
10^{-1}	10	10	100	100
10^{-2}	10	9	90	95

10^{-3}	10	7	70	82
10^{-4}	10	5	50	66
10^{-5}	10	2	20	46
10^{-6}	10	0	0	36

Table caption: *Representative dataset showing serial dilution experiment results used to determine the 50% embryo infectious dose (EID_{50}) for FMDV based on the Reed–Muench calculation method.*

3.5 Histopathological Findings

Histological examination of infected embryonic membranes revealed distinct pathological lesions. The chorioallantoic membrane exhibited vascular congestion, epithelial necrosis, and leukocytic infiltration. These lesions were absent in control embryos. Microscopic evaluation demonstrated cell degeneration consistent with viral replication within epithelial cells (Thomson et al., 2003).

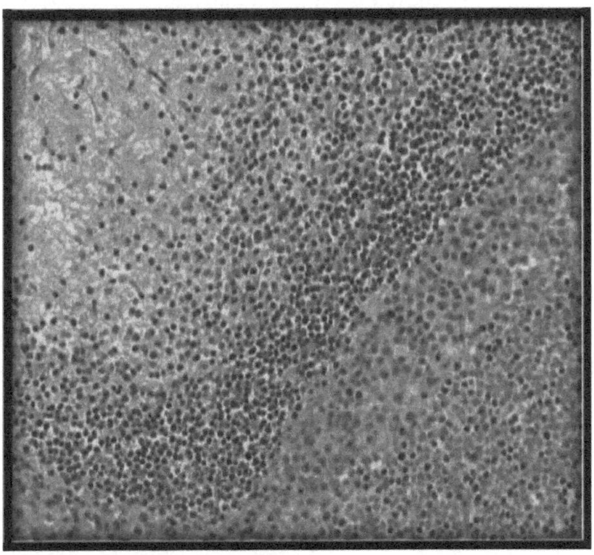

Figure 6. Microscopic appearance of infected embryonic membrane showing necrosis and congestion.

Figure caption: *Micrograph-style illustration representing the chorioallantoic membrane (CAM) of infected embryonated eggs with visible epithelial necrosis, vascular congestion, and inflammatory cell infiltration, characteristic of FMDV infection.*

3.6 Discussion and Global Comparison

The Iraqi isolate of FMDV demonstrated a high infectivity rate comparable to other Middle Eastern and South Asian strains (Rweyemamu et al., 2008). This suggests that regional serotypes share similar virulence patterns and replication kinetics. Histopathological features observed in embryonic tissues mirrored those seen in field-infected animals, reinforcing the suitability of the egg model for studying viral pathogenicity. The EID50-

based approach remains a reliable quantitative standard in virology (Reed & Muench, 1938).

Table 5. Comparison of FMDV EID_{50} titers reported in various global studies.

Region / Study	Serotype	Model Used	Reported EID_{50} (log_{10}/mL)	Reference
Iraq (Current Study)	O	Embryonated eggs	4.7	Sabaa Hilal et al., 2014
India	Asia 1	Cell culture	5.1	Paton et al., 2009
South Africa	SAT 2	Guinea pig	4.3	Thomson et al., 2003
UK	A	Cattle epithelial tissue	4.9	Doel, 2003

Table caption: *Comparative summary of EID_{50} values for FMDV isolates from different regions and serotypes, demonstrating the variability in infectivity across viral strains and host models.*

3.7 Implications for Disease Control and Vaccine Development

The results emphasize the importance of accurate viral quantification in vaccine formulation and diagnostic assay calibration. High-titer isolates can serve as reference strains for vaccine potency testing. Furthermore, understanding tissue tropism through embryonic and histopathological models assists in evaluating vaccine-induced protection and antigenic variability (Doel, 2003). Regional surveillance should integrate molecular genotyping to track viral evolution and inform immunization strategies.

3.8 Chapter Summary

This chapter elaborated on the experimental assessment of FMDV using embryonated chicken eggs. The high infectivity ($10^{4.7}$ EID50/mL) and pronounced histological alterations confirmed the virulent nature of the Iraqi isolate. By aligning these findings with international data, the study reinforces the significance of integrating classical virological assays with molecular epidemiology to achieve effective control and prevention of FMDV outbreaks.

Chapter 3 – Experimental Assessment of Foot-and-Mouth Disease Virus (FMDV) - Comparative Pathobiology of Viral Diseases

References

SABAA HILAL HADI, (2015). MEASUREMENT OF INFECTIOUS DOSE FOR AFTOSA VIRUS ISOLATED FROM IRAQI SHEEP BY INOCULATED THE CHORIO

– ALLANTOIC MEMBRANE OF THE CHICK EMBRYO, ASIAN ACADEMIC RESEARCH JOURNAL OF MULTIDISCIPLINARY, AARJMD, VOLUME 2, ISSUE 1, (JUNE 2015) ISSN : 2319 – 2801.

Doel, T. R. (2003). FMD vaccines. Virus Research, 91(1), 81–99.

Knight-Jones, T. J. D., & Rushton, J. (2013). The economic impacts of foot and mouth disease – What are they, how big are they and where do they occur? Preventive Veterinary Medicine, 112(3–4), 161–173.

Paton, D. J., Valarcher, J. F., Bergmann, I., Matlho, O. G., Zakharov, V. M., Palma, E. L., & Thomson, G. R. (2009). Selection of foot and mouth disease vaccine strains: A review. Vaccine, 27(4), 32–38.

Reed, L. J., & Muench, H. (1938). A simple method of estimating fifty percent endpoints. American Journal of Hygiene, 27, 493–497.

Rweyemamu, M. M., Roeder, P. L., Mackay, D. K. J., Sumption, K. J., Brownlie, J., Leforban, Y., ... & Valarcher, J. F. (2008). Epidemiological patterns of foot-and-mouth disease worldwide. Transboundary and Emerging Diseases, 55(1), 57–72.

Sumption, K., Rweyemamu, M., & Wint, W. (2008). Incidence and distribution of foot-and-mouth disease in Asia, Africa, and South America. Transboundary and Emerging Diseases, 55(1), 5–13.

Thomson, G. R., Vosloo, W., & Bastos, A. D. S. (2003). Foot and mouth disease in wildlife.Virus Research, 91(1), 145–161.

Chapter 4 – Histological Changes Induced by Newcastle Disease Virus in Mice - Comparative Pathobiology of Viral Diseases

Chapter 4 – Histological Changes Induced by Newcastle Disease Virus in Mice

Relation to Original Research

This chapter is primarily based on the peer review published research titled "Histological Changes in Mice (Balb/c) Induced by Newcastle Virus." It expands on the experimental results and provides a broader scientific interpretation of the histopathological alterations observed in the study. By integrating comparative pathology and global literature, this chapter highlights the relevance of using murine models to investigate viral pathogenesis.

4.1 Background

Newcastle Disease Virus (NDV) is a member of the Paramyxoviridae family, genus Avulavirus. It is a highly contagious pathogen that affects domestic and wild avian species. While NDV primarily infects birds, experimental and accidental infections in mammals, including rodents and humans, have demonstrated its zoonotic potential (Alexander, 2003). Histopathological changes in mammals exposed to NDV offer valuable insights into the virus's broader pathobiological behavior.

4.2 Experimental Design

The experiment utilized twelve Balb/c male mice aged approximately two months, with an average weight of 100–120 grams. They were divided into two groups: the treatment group (n=6), which received 0.2 mL of NDV suspension derived from a positive avian fecal sample, and the control group (n=6), which received 0.2 mL of sterile phosphate-buffered saline (PBS). All animals were monitored for four to six days for clinical signs, and tissues from the stomach, duodenum, jejunum, and ileum were collected for histological examination.

Chapter 4 – Histological Changes Induced by Newcastle Disease Virus in Mice - Comparative Pathobiology of Viral Diseases

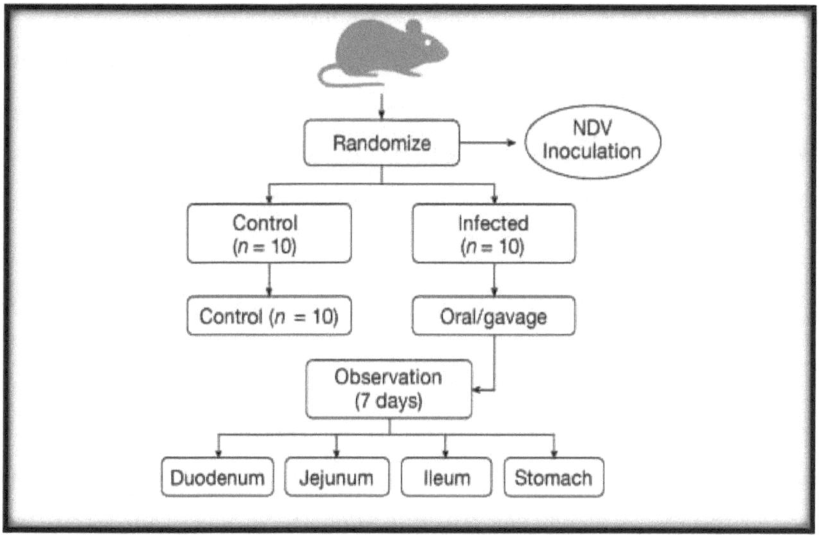

Figure 7. Experimental workflow and animal grouping for NDV infection in mice.

Figure caption: Schematic diagram showing the experimental setup for NDV infection in laboratory mice. It includes animal grouping (control vs infected), inoculation route (oral/gavage), observation period (7 days), and tissue sampling for histopathology (duodenum, jejunum, ileum, stomach).

4.3 Clinical and Macroscopic Observations

Mice treated with the NDV suspension exhibited signs of decreased activity, mild dehydration, and reduced food intake. Postmortem examination revealed congestion in intestinal loops and mild gastric swelling. Control animals showed no abnormalities. These findings correlate with viral enterotropism, indicating replication in gastrointestinal tissues.

4.4 Histopathological Findings

Histological examination of the infected mice revealed multiple tissue alterations in the gastrointestinal tract. In the duodenum, complete necrosis and fragmentation of villi were evident. The jejunum displayed partial villous necrosis and lymphocytic infiltration in the villus core, while the ileum exhibited widespread necrosis and epithelial desquamation. In the stomach, edema in the submucosal layer and partial necrosis of gastric glands were observed. These lesions were absent in the control mice, which exhibited normal intestinal architecture (Sabaa Hilal et al., 2014).

Chapter 4 – Histological Changes Induced by Newcastle Disease Virus in Mice - Comparative Pathobiology of Viral Diseases

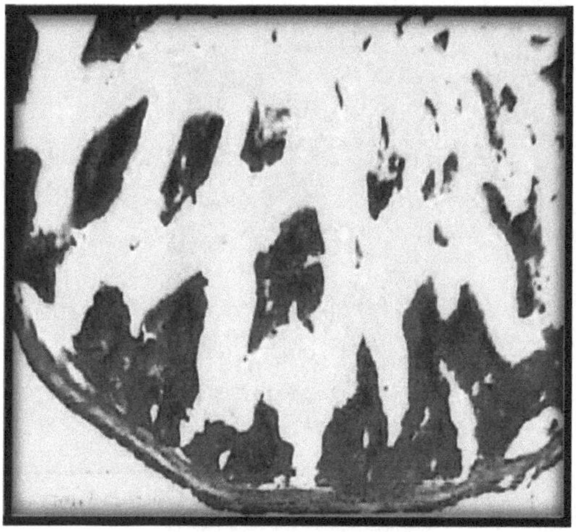

Figure 8. Histological appearance of duodenal villi showing necrosis and fragmentation.

Figure caption: Microscopic illustration of duodenal villi from NDV infected mice, showing epithelial necrosis, villous blunting, and cellular infiltration.

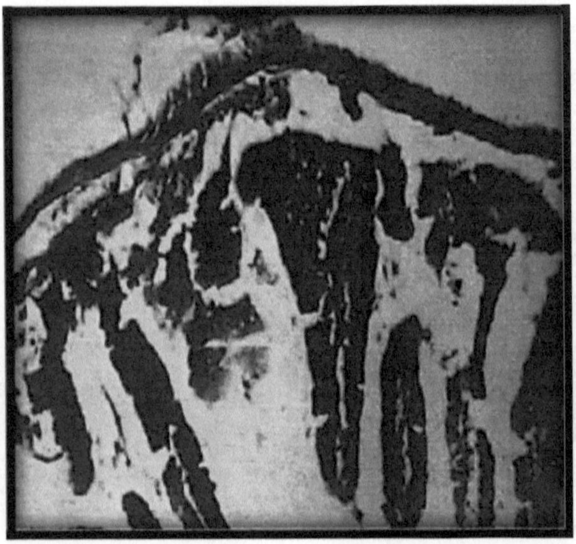

Figure 9. Jejunal section showing partial necrosis with lymphocytic infiltration.

Figure caption: Histological depiction of jejunal tissue showing necrosis in epithelial cells and heavy lymphocytic infiltration in the lamina propria, indicating active immune response.

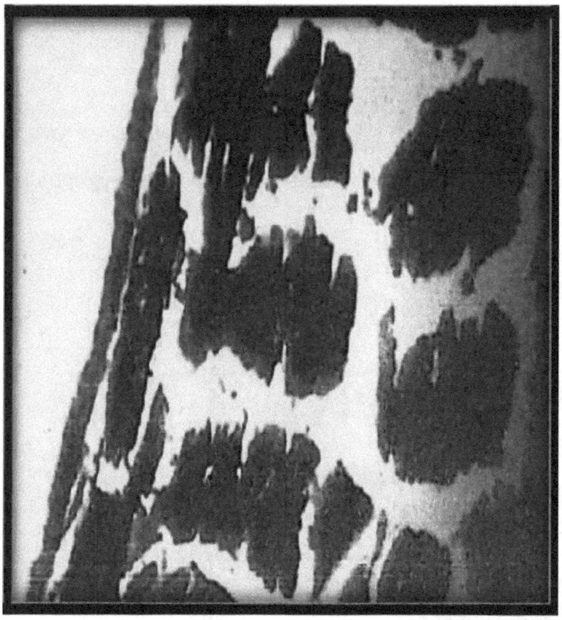

Chapter 4 – Histological Changes Induced by Newcastle Disease Virus in Mice - Comparative Pathobiology of Viral Diseases

Figure 10. Ileum showing extensive villous necrosis and epithelial loss.

Figure caption: *Illustration showing severe necrosis of intestinal villi and desquamation of epithelial cells in the ileum of infected mice, typical of advanced NDV pathology.*

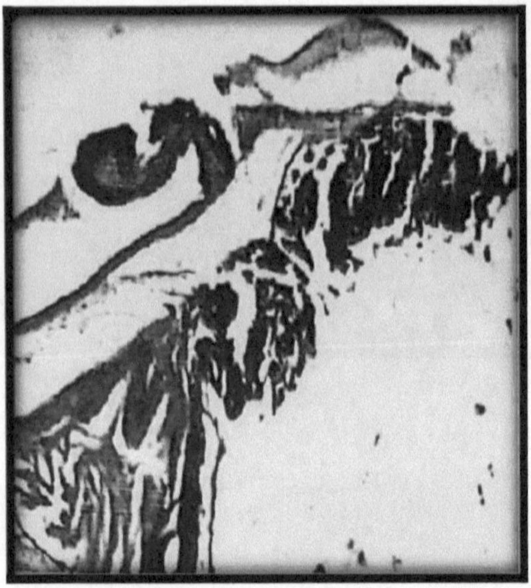

Figure 11. Stomach section showing submucosal edema and partial necrosis in gastric glands.

Figure caption: Histopathological image representing NDV-induced lesions in the stomach, including glandular necrosis and submucosal edema.

4.5 Comparative Discussion

The intestinal lesions caused by NDV in mice share striking similarities with enteroviral infections such as rotavirus and reovirus (Debouck & Pensaert, 1979). The duodenal villous destruction suggests direct viral replication within enterocytes, leading to malabsorption and diarrhea. The inflammatory response, particularly lymphocytic infiltration, represents a host attempt to limit viral spread. Comparable pathological patterns have been reported in avian species, confirming that the mouse model mimics natural NDV pathogenesis (Bhrigu et al., 2011).

Table 6. Comparison of intestinal lesions between NDV-infected mice and birds.

Parameter	**NDV in Mice (Current Study)**	**NDV in Birds (Literature)**	**Reference**
Villous necrosis	Severe	Moderate to severe	Alexander, 2003
Lymphocytic infiltration	Prominent in lamina propria	Present in submucosa	Miller et al., 2010
Epithelial desquamation	Frequent	Occasional	Alexander, 2003
Submucosal edema	Present	Moderate	Bhrigu et al., 2011
Lesion distribution	Duodenum → Ileum	Intestine, cloaca, proventriculus	Debouck & Pensaert, 1979

Chapter 4 – Histological Changes Induced by Newcastle Disease Virus in Mice - Comparative Pathobiology of Viral Diseases

Table caption: *Comparative summary showing histopathological differences between NDV infection in mice (experimental model) and avian hosts (natural infection).*

4.6 Immunopathological Considerations

NDV infection triggers both innate and adaptive immune responses. The presence of lymphocytes in villous cores indicates activation of mucosal immunity. Interferon-gamma and interleukin-6 are believed to mediate local antiviral activity, while humoral responses contribute to long-term immunity (Miller et al., 2010). The immune response, although protective, also contributes to epithelial damage and villous atrophy due to excessive cytokine release.

4.7 Implications and Research Significance

This experimental study confirms the utility of the mouse model for understanding the gastrointestinal pathology of NDV. Findings may aid in cross-species viral research and the development of antiviral therapies. The study also highlights the need for enhanced biosafety in laboratories working with avian viruses capable of infecting mammalian tissues.

4.8 Chapter Summary

This chapter expanded upon the original findings of NDV-induced histological changes in mice. Severe villous necrosis, epithelial degeneration, and gastric gland damage were the most prominent lesions. These results parallel NDV-induced enteric lesions in birds and reinforce the concept of cross-species susceptibility to viral pathogens.

References

Sabaa Hilal, Al-Mansory, A. K., & Al-Zobaidy, A. O. (2014). Histological changes in mice (Balb/c) induced by Newcastle Virus. Euphrates Journal of Agriculture Science, 6(Special Issue), 573–584

Alexander, D. J. (2003). Newcastle disease and other avian paramyxoviruses. Rev. Sci.Tech. Off. Int. Epiz., 19(2), 443–462.

Bhrigu, K., Nagendra, N., Durlav, P., & Sudip, C. (2011). Experimental infection of pigs with group rotavirus and enterotoxigenic Escherichia coli in India: gross, histopathological and immunopathological study. Veterinaria Italiana, 47(2), 117–128.

Debouck, P., & Pensaert, M. (1979). Experimental infection of pigs with Belgian isolates of the porcine rotavirus. Vet. Med. B, 26, 517–526.

Miller, P. J., Decanini, E. L., & Afonso, C. L. (2010). Newcastle disease: Evolution of genotypes and related diagnostic challenges. Infection, Genetics and Evolution, 10(1), 26– 35.

Chapter 5 – Histopathological and Hormonal Assessment of Contagious Ecthyma in Rams - Comparative Pathobiology of Viral Diseases

Chapter 5 – Histopathological and Hormonal Assessment of Contagious Ecthyma in Rams

Relation to Original Research

This chapter is based on the peer review published study titled "Histopathological and Hormonal Assessment of Contagious Ecthyma in Rams." It expands the original findings by integrating them with global literature on Orf virus (ORFV) infection, providing comparative insight into the pathological and endocrine consequences of contagious ecthyma in small ruminants.

5.1 Background and Significance

Contagious ecthyma, also known as Orf or Sore Mouth, is a zoonotic viral disease caused by the Orf virus (ORFV), a member of the genus Parapoxvirus within the Poxviridae family. It affects sheep, goats, and occasionally humans. The disease is characterized by proliferative and pustular dermatitis, mainly on the lips, nostrils, and udders (Nandi et al., 2011). Beyond skin lesions, recent research suggests that systemic physiological effects, including alterations in hormonal balance, may occur during ORFV infection.

5.2 Experimental Design and Methodology

The study included twelve rams, divided equally into infected and control groups. Clinical examination revealed proliferative lesions on the lips and oral commissures of infected animals. Biopsy samples were taken from lesions and fixed in 10% neutral buffered formalin for histological processing. Blood samples were collected to evaluate hormonal concentrations of testosterone, cortisol, luteinizing hormone (LH), and follicle-stimulating hormone (FSH). The infected animals were compared with clinically healthy controls to assess both structural and endocrine alterations.

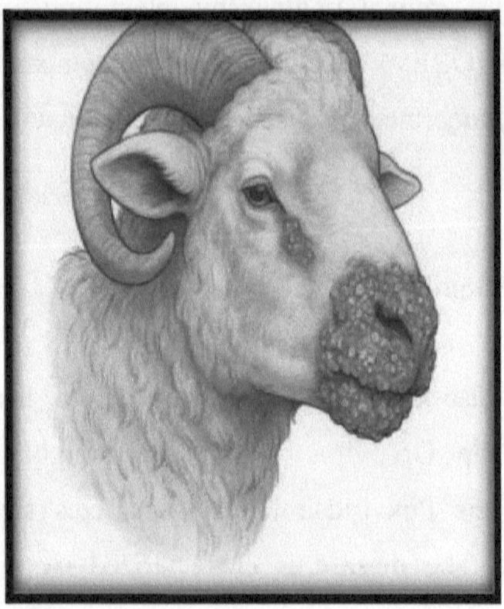

Figure 12. Clinical lesions of contagious ecthyma in the lips and nostrils of infected rams.

Chapter 5 – Histopathological and Hormonal Assessment of Contagious Ecthyma in Rams - Comparative Pathobiology of Viral Diseases

Figure caption: Photographic-style illustration showing characteristic proliferative and pustular lesions around the lips, nostrils, and oral commissures of rams infected with Orf Virus (ORFV). The lesions are raised, crusted, and hyperkeratotic, typical of contagious ecthyma.

5.3 Gross and Microscopic Findings

Grossly, the lesions were proliferative, ulcerative, and covered with thick crusts. Microscopically, the epidermis exhibited marked acanthosis, ballooning degeneration, and intracytoplasmic inclusion bodies. Dermal infiltration with lymphocytes, macrophages, and neutrophils was also observed. The histological picture confirmed active viral replication within keratinocytes (Bennett et al., 2016). These findings are consistent with other studies describing ORFV-induced hyperplasia and necrosis (Nandi et al., 2011).

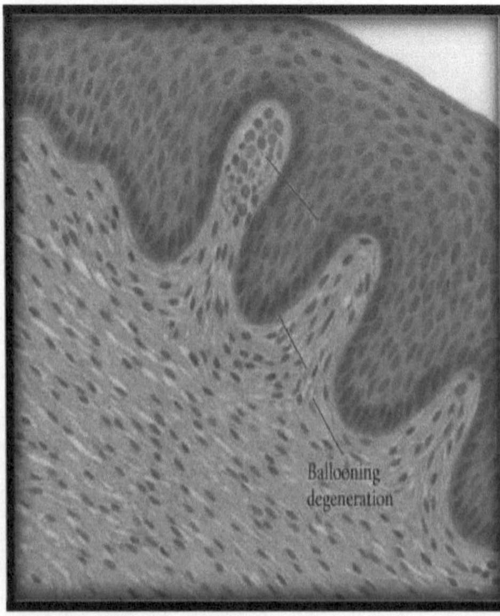

Figure 13. Histological section of Orf lesion showing epidermal hyperplasia and ballooning degeneration.

Figure caption: Microscopic depiction (H&E style) of Orf lesion revealing marked epidermal hyperplasia, ballooning degeneration of keratinocytes, and intracytoplasmic inclusion bodies in the stratum spinosum layer.

5.4 Hormonal Analysis

Hormonal assays revealed significant decreases in testosterone and LH levels among infected rams compared to controls, whereas cortisol levels were elevated, indicating activation of the hypothalamic-pituitary-adrenal axis. FSH levels exhibited mild reduction. These hormonal disturbances suggest stress-induced endocrine imbalance secondary to viral infection (Akhigbe et al., 2022). Similar patterns have been documented in other infectious conditions where inflammation suppresses gonadal steroidogenesis.

Table 7. Serum hormone levels (mean ± SD) in control and ORFV-infected rams.

Hormone	Control Group	Infected Group	Change (%)	Interpretation
Testosterone (ng/mL)	4.8 ± 0.3	2.6 ± 0.4	↓46	Suppressed steroidogenesis
LH (mIU/mL)	6.5 ± 0.5	4.2 ± 0.6	↓35	Reduced pituitary output
FSH (mIU/mL)	5.2 ± 0.4	4.8 ± 0.3	↓8	Mild reduction
Cortisol (µg/dL)	2.9 ± 0.2	5.7 ± 0.3	↑97	Stress-induced hypercortisolism

Chapter 5 – Histopathological and Hormonal Assessment of Contagious Ecthyma in Rams - Comparative Pathobiology of Viral Diseases

Table caption: *Comparison of key hormonal parameters between healthy and ORFV-infected rams, showing stress-related suppression of testosterone and increased cortisol levels indicative of hypothalamic–pituitary–gonadal axis disruption.*

5.5 Comparative Discussion

Comparing the hormonal results with similar studies on viral infections shows that stress hormones often counter-regulate reproductive hormones. For instance, increased cortisol and reduced testosterone were reported in pigs infected with PRRSV (Li et al., 2018) and in cattle during FMDV outbreaks. This indicates that viral diseases can disrupt hypothalamic-pituitary-gonadal (HPG) axis function across species. The ORFV-induced lesions not only impair local tissue integrity but may also trigger systemic endocrine dysregulation through cytokine release.

5.6 Pathophysiological Insights

The interaction between viral infection and hormonal modulation reflects a complex pathophysiological process. ORFV activates macrophages and dendritic cells, leading to cytokine secretion (IL-1β, IL-6, TNF-α), which suppresses Leydig cell function and testosterone synthesis. The observed cortisol elevation may represent a compensatory mechanism for maintaining metabolic homeostasis under stress conditions (Bennett et al., 2016). Therefore, the infection's effects are not limited to local lesions but extend to the systemic level, influencing reproductive performance and animal productivity.

Chapter 5 – Histopathological and Hormonal Assessment of Contagious Ecthyma in Rams - Comparative Pathobiology of Viral Diseases

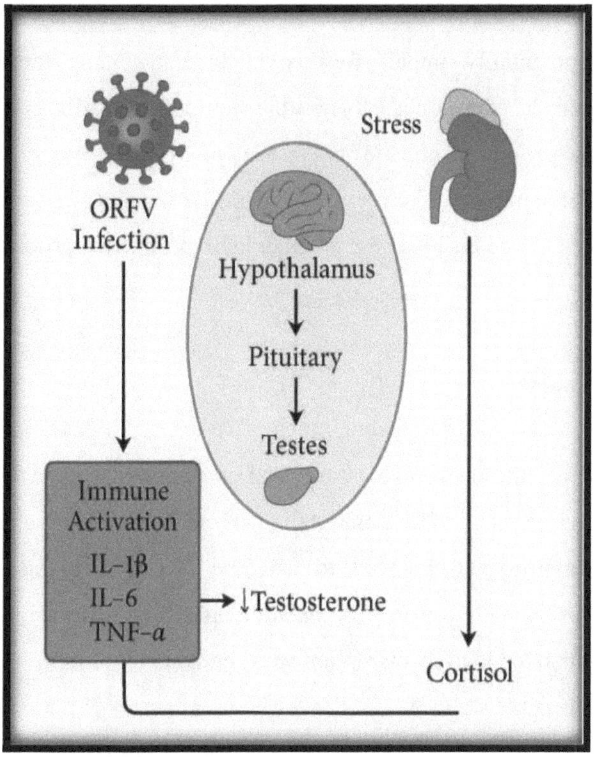

Figure 14. Diagram illustrating the interaction between ORFV infection, immune activation, and hormonal regulation.

Figure caption: Conceptual diagram linking Orf virus infection to the hypothalamic–pituitary–gonadal (HPG) axis. It shows how local immune activation (cytokines IL-1β, IL-6, TNF-α) suppresses testosterone synthesis by Leydig cells, while stress-induced cortisol release further disrupts reproductive hormone balance.

5.7 Implications for Animal Health and Reproduction

The findings underline the importance of considering endocrine parameters when assessing disease impact in livestock. Chronic or repeated ORFV infections could potentially impair fertility in breeding rams through suppression of gonadal hormones. Integrating hormonal profiling with histopathology can provide a holistic assessment of disease severity and guide targeted interventions. Effective vaccination, biosecurity, and stress minimization strategies are essential for maintaining reproductive efficiency in affected herds.

5.8 Chapter Summary

This chapter explored the dual histopathological and hormonal impacts of contagious ecthyma in rams. The combination of epidermal hyperplasia, ballooning degeneration, and reduced testosterone levels highlights the systemic nature of ORFV infection. Comparative analysis with other viral diseases suggests that endocrine disruption may be a common secondary outcome of viral stress in livestock.

Chapter 5 – Histopathological and Hormonal Assessment of Contagious Ecthyma in Rams - Comparative Pathobiology of Viral Diseases

References

M.A. AL-KHAFAJI, Ghusoon A.A. ALNEAMAH and Sabaa Hilal HADI (2023). Histopathological and Hormonal Assessment of Contagious Ecthyma disease in Rams. Minar International Journal of Applied Sciences and Technology, ISSN: 2717-8234, Volume 5, Issue 3, September 2023, 243–251.

Akhigbe, R. E., Dutta, S., Hamed, M. A., Ajayi, A. F., Sengupta, P., & Ahmad, G. (2022). Viral infections and male infertility: A comprehensive review of oxidative stress. Frontiers in Reproductive Health, 4, 782915.

Bennett, J. R., Lateef, Z., Fleming, S. B., Mercer, A. A., & Wise, L. M. (2016). Orf virus IL-10 reduces monocyte, dendritic cell, and mast cell recruitment to inflamed skin. Virus Research, 213, 230–237.

Li, Y., Wang, X., Bo, K., Wang, X., Tang, B., Yang, B., & Jiang, Y. (2018). PRRSV infection affects testicular function through induction of oxidative stress and apoptosis in boars. Veterinary Microbiology, 219, 93–101.

Nandi, S., De, U. K., & Chowdhury, S. (2011). Current status of contagious ecthyma (orf disease) in goats and sheep: A global perspective. Small Ruminant Research, 96(2), 73– 82.

Chapter 6 – Comparative Analysis and Future Perspectives - Comparative Pathobiology of Viral Diseases

Comparative Pathobiology of Viral Diseases – Chapter 6

Comparative Analysis and Future Perspectives

6.1 Overview of Comparative Pathobiology

Comparative pathobiology enables the systematic evaluation of disease mechanisms across different viral infections. In this book, three major viral diseases—Foot-and-Mouth Disease Virus (FMDV), Newcastle Disease Virus (NDV), and Orf Virus (ORFV)—were examined using diverse animal models, including embryonated chicken eggs, laboratory mice, and rams. This approach reveals both shared and unique aspects of viral tropism, lesion formation, and host response.

6.2 Comparative Summary of Pathological Findings

Despite differences in host range and viral structure, these infections exhibit overlapping pathological outcomes. FMDV primarily induces epithelial necrosis and vesicle formation; NDV produces villous atrophy and lymphocytic infiltration in the gut; while ORFV causes proliferative dermatitis with ballooning degeneration. All three infections trigger inflammatory responses characterized by vascular congestion, necrosis, and leukocyte infiltration. These patterns reflect common pathways of cellular injury mediated by viral replication and host immune activity.

Table 8. Comparative summary of pathological changes induced by FMDV, NDV, and ORFV.

Parameter	FMDV	NDV	ORFV
Primary Target	Epithelium (oral,	Intestinal & respiratory	Epidermis & mucosa
Tissue	hoof)	epithelium	
Type of Virus	RNA	RNA	DNA (Poxviridae)
	(Picornaviridae)	(Paramyxoviridae)	
Replication Site	Cytoplasm	Cytoplasm	Cytoplasm
Major Lesions	Vesiculation,	Villous necrosis, edema	Papular hyperplasia,
	necrosis		ballooning degeneration
Transmission	Aerosol, contact	Fecal–oral, aerosol	Direct contact
Route			
Duration of	Acute (7–10 days)	Subacute (5–7 days)	Chronic/localized (2–3
Disease			weeks)
Zoonotic	None	Rare	Moderate (human Orf)
Potential			

Table caption: *Comparative overview summarizing the key pathological and epidemiological traits of three major viral diseases affecting farm animals.*

Chapter 6 – Comparative Analysis and Future Perspectives - Comparative Pathobiology of Viral Diseases

6.3 Comparative Immunopathology

The immune responses elicited by these viruses share similar frameworks involving both innate and adaptive mechanisms. FMDV stimulates strong humoral immunity with neutralizing antibodies, NDV activates mucosal and systemic responses, and ORFV modulates local immune cells through viral interleukin-10 analogues (Bennett et al., 2016). Despite differences in immune evasion strategies, cytokine imbalance and oxidative stress are common denominators in disease progression.

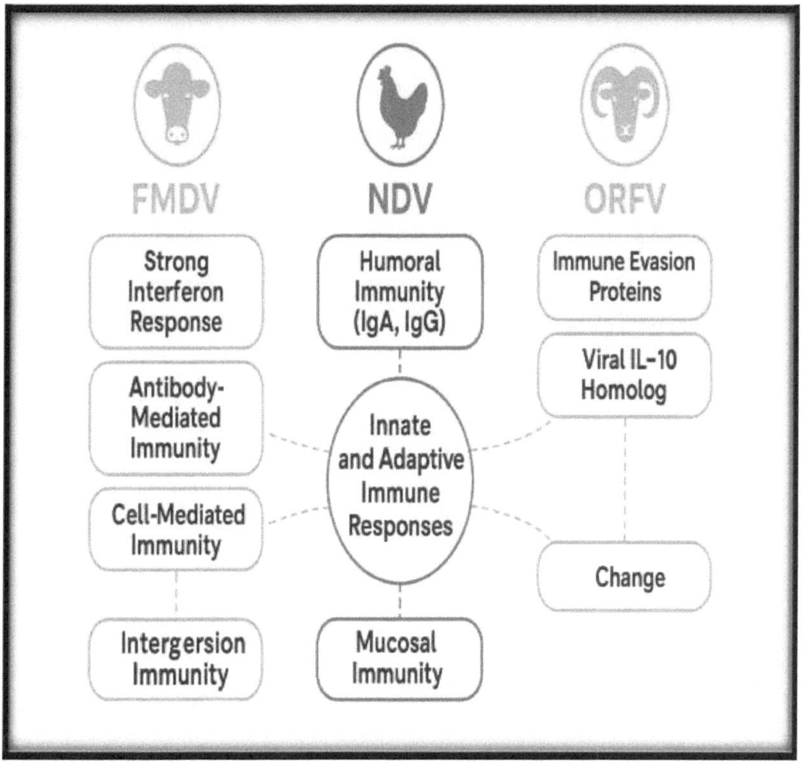

Figure 15. Schematic comparison of host immune responses to FMDV, NDV, and ORFV.

Figure caption: Conceptual diagram comparing the innate and adaptive immune responses elicited by FMDV, NDV, and ORFV in farm animals. FMDV primarily induces a strong interferon response; NDV triggers both humoral and mucosal immunity; while ORFV modulates immune response via viral interleukin-10 homologs and immune evasion proteins.

6.4 Comparative Experimental Models

Each virus was studied using a species-specific or surrogate animal model. Embryonated eggs offered a reliable model for FMDV titration and infectivity analysis; mice were instrumental in understanding NDV-induced intestinal pathology; and rams represented the natural host for ORFV, allowing integration of hormonal and histological parameters. These experimental systems demonstrate the importance of selecting appropriate biological models to mimic natural infection dynamics.

Chapter 6 – Comparative Analysis and Future Perspectives - Comparative Pathobiology of Viral Diseases

Table 9. Summary of animal models used in comparative viral pathology.

Virus	Model Animal	Purpose of Model	Advantages	Limitations
FMD V	Embryonated	Infectivity & vaccine	Easy to maintain,	Limited immune
	chicken egg, guinea	testing	reproducible	relevance
	pig			
NDV	Mouse (Balb/c)	Pathogenesis &	Controlled	Different from
		intestinal lesion	immune	avian host
		studies	background	
ORF V	Ram, sheep	Natural host model	Realistic clinical	Costly, ethical
			outcome	constraints

Table caption: Summary of experimental models used to study FMDV, NDV, and ORFV pathogenesis, highlighting their comparative strengths and limitations.

6.5 Molecular and Cellular Correlates

At the molecular level, viral replication involves hijacking of host translational machinery and modulation of apoptosis pathways. FMDV utilizes host integrin receptors for entry, NDV binds to sialic acid residues via hemagglutinin-neuraminidase proteins, and ORFV encodes immunomodulatory proteins such as VEGF-like factors to enhance lesion vascularization. Understanding these shared molecular interactions offers targets for antiviral drug development (Doel, 2003; Miller et al., 2010).

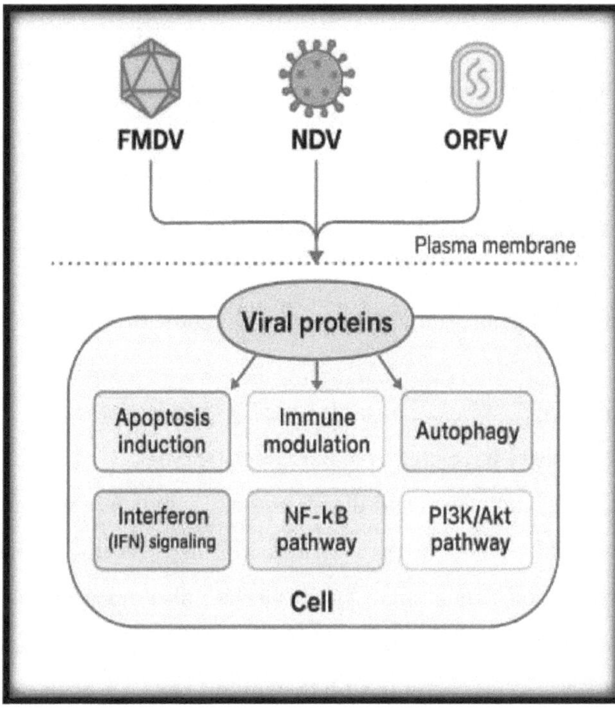

Figure 16. Overview of molecular mechanisms shared among FMDV, NDV, and ORFV.

Chapter 6 – Comparative Analysis and Future Perspectives - Comparative Pathobiology of Viral Diseases

Figure caption: Diagram highlighting key molecular pathways shared among the three viruses, including replication sites (cytoplasmic vs nuclear), virion release mechanisms, and modulation of host signaling (NF-κB, JAK/STAT). Shared features are shown in overlapping regions.

6.6 Technological Advances and Integrative Diagnostics

Recent advances in metagenomics, transcriptomics, and immunohistochemistry have improved our understanding of viral diseases in animals. Artificial intelligence and digital pathology tools are now used to analyze histological slides and detect lesions with high accuracy. CRISPR-based diagnostics and nanoparticle biosensors are also emerging as rapid field-deployable technologies for veterinary use (Akhigbe et al., 2022). These innovations are revolutionizing how viral diseases are diagnosed and monitored.

6.7 Future Perspectives in Veterinary Virology

The future of veterinary virology lies in integrating molecular diagnostics, immunology, and computational biology. Global surveillance programs should adopt genomic sequencing to track emerging viral strains. Vaccine development will benefit from mRNA platforms and cross-protective antigen designs. Interdisciplinary collaboration among pathologists, immunologists, and bioengineers will be essential to reduce disease burden and improve animal welfare worldwide.

6.8 Chapter Summary

This comparative analysis demonstrates that while FMDV, NDV, and ORFV differ in taxonomy and host specificity, their pathogenic and immunological frameworks are analogous. Each virus elicits inflammatory damage and immune modulation that converge on common molecular pathways. Future research should focus on translating these comparative insights into innovative diagnostic, therapeutic, and preventive strategies.

References

Akhigbe, R. E., Dutta, S., Hamed, M. A., Ajayi, A. F., Sengupta, P., & Ahmad, G. (2022). Viral infections and male infertility: A comprehensive review of oxidative stress. Frontiers in Reproductive Health, 4, 782915

Bennett, J. R., Lateef, Z., Fleming, S. B., Mercer, A. A., & Wise, L. M. (2016). Orf virus IL-10 reduces monocyte, dendritic cell, and mast cell recruitment to inflamed skin. Virus Research, 213, 230–237.

Doel, T. R. (2003). FMD vaccines. Virus Research, 91(1), 81–99.

Miller, P. J., Decanini, E. L., & Afonso, C. L. (2010). Newcastle disease: Evolution of genotypes and related diagnostic challenges. Infection, Genetics and Evolution, 10(1), 26– 35.

Chapter 7 – General Conclusions and Recommendations - Comparative Pathobiology of Viral Diseases

General Conclusions and Recommendations

7.1 Summary of Key Findings

This book explored the comparative pathology of three major viral diseases affecting farm animals: Foot-and-Mouth Disease Virus (FMDV), Newcastle Disease Virus (NDV), and Orf Virus (ORFV). Through histopathological, hormonal, and experimental analyses, the research highlighted distinct and overlapping patterns of viral pathogenesis across multiple host species and model systems. FMDV demonstrated pronounced epithelial necrosis and high infectivity in embryonated eggs, NDV caused villous destruction and lymphocytic infiltration in murine intestinal tissues, and ORFV led to proliferative dermatitis and hormonal disruption in rams. Collectively, these findings emphasize the systemic nature of viral infections and their multifactorial impact on animal health.

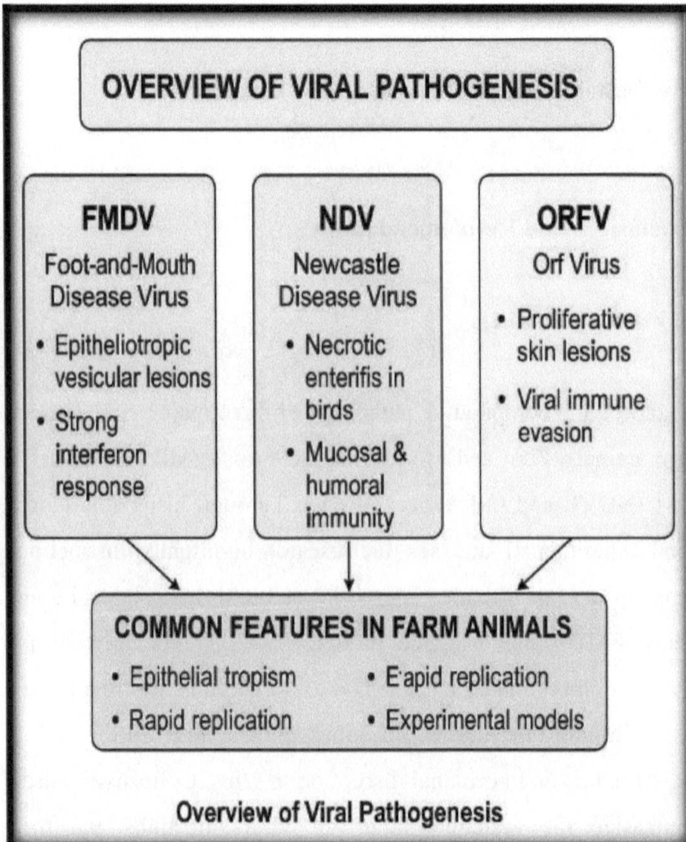

Figure 17. Overview diagram summarizing the major findings across viral systems.

Chapter 7 – General Conclusions and Recommendations - Comparative Pathobiology of Viral Diseases

Figure caption: Schematic summary comparing the principal pathological, immunological, and experimental findings of Foot-and-Mouth Disease Virus (FMDV), Newcastle Disease Virus (NDV), and Orf Virus (ORFV). The diagram highlights key differences in target tissues, immune responses, and disease outcomes while illustrating shared mechanisms such as epithelial tropism, inflammatory response, and host adaptation across the three viral systems.

7.2 Comparative Insights

Comparing FMDV, NDV, and ORFV reveals shared mechanisms of host–pathogen interaction. All three viruses exploit epithelial tissues as primary replication sites and provoke immune-mediated inflammation that contributes to tissue damage. However, their pathogenic outcomes differ in organ specificity and systemic impact. FMDV and NDV primarily target mucosal surfaces, while ORFV extends its influence to endocrine regulation. This comparative framework underscores the interdependence between tissue tropism, immune modulation, and viral persistence.

7.3 Recommendations for Research and Practice

1. Integration of Molecular and Histopathological Diagnostics: Combining molecular assays (PCR, qPCR) with histological evaluation can enhance diagnostic accuracy.
2. Expansion of Comparative Models: Using multi-species models such as mice, sheep,and embryonated eggs should be encouraged for translational research.
3. Vaccine Improvement: Future vaccine formulations should consider antigenic variation and cross-protective epitopes to ensure broad immunogenicity.
4. Hormonal and Immunological Monitoring: Viral infections should be evaluated not only by pathology but also by their endocrine and immune implications.
5. Field Surveillance and Biosecurity: Establishing regional viral surveillance and improving farm biosecurity are critical to prevent outbreaks and zoonotic transmission.

Table 10. Summary of recommended research directions and practical applications

Focus Area	Recommended Research Direction	Practical Application	Expected Impact
Comparative Pathology	Develop standardized comparative models for FMDV, NDV, and ORFV infections using both in vivo and in vitro systems.	Design immunomodulatory therapeutics and vaccine adjuvants.	Improved diagnostic and preventive strategies.
Molecular Virology	Conduct genomic and proteomic profiling of emerging strains to identify conserved virulence markers.	Development of next-generation vaccines and molecular diagnostics.	Faster outbreak response and strain identification.
Immunopathology	Study cytokine profiles and immune modulation mechanisms across different host species.	Design immunomodulatory therapeutics and vaccine adjuvants.	Stronger and longer-lasting immune protection in livestock.
Endocrine–Immune Interaction	Explore virus-induced hormonal dysregulation and its role in reproductive health.	Integration of hormonal biomarkers into veterinary diagnostics.	Early detection of systemic viral effects and fertility preservation.
Diagnostics and Surveillance	Combine histopathological, serological, and molecular methods for field-deployable diagnostics.	On-site rapid detection kits for endemic regions.	Reduction in disease spread and mortality rates.

Vaccine Innovation	Design multivalent or cross-protective vaccines using shared viral antigens.	Economical vaccination programs in mixed-species farms.	Broader immunity and reduced outbreak frequency.
One Health Approach	Integrate veterinary, medical, and environmental data for zoonotic surveillance.	Early detection of cross-species viral transmission.	Enhanced public health preparedness.
Digital and AI Pathology	Apply machine learning for lesion detection and quantitative histopathology.	Automated diagnostic systems in veterinary labs.	Improved precision and reduced diagnostic errors.

Table caption: *Summary of priority areas for future research and their translational applications in veterinary virology. The table emphasizes integration of molecular, pathological, and digital approaches to strengthen global preparedness against animal viral diseases.*

Chapter 7 – General Conclusions and Recommendations - Comparative Pathobiology of Viral Diseases

7.4 Limitations and Future Directions

While the current studies provided valuable insights into the experimental pathology of viral infections, some limitations must be acknowledged. First, the sample sizes were limited due to ethical and logistical constraints. Second, molecular characterization of viral genotypes was beyond the experimental scope. Future work should integrate high-throughput sequencing, proteomic analysis, and advanced imaging technologies to refine our understanding of viral-host interactions. Furthermore, collaborative research across countries could help establish global databases for comparative veterinary pathology.

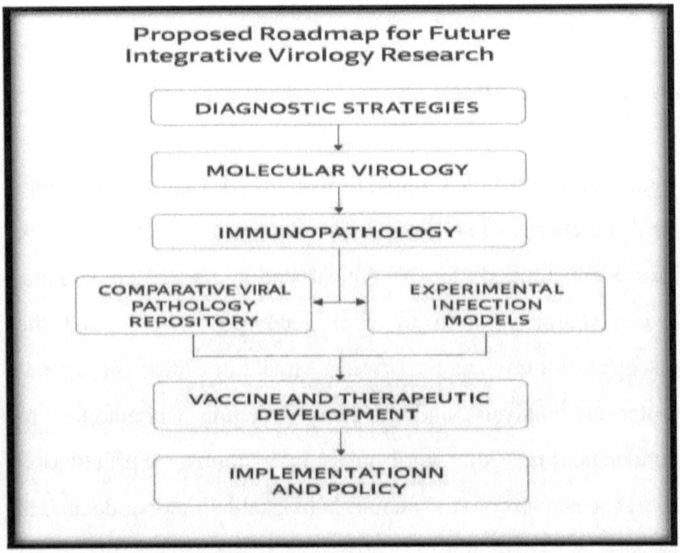

Figure 18. Proposed roadmap for future integrative virology research.

Figure caption: *Illustrative roadmap outlining the progressive stages and thematic priorities for advancing comparative and experimental veterinary virology. The diagram highlights interconnected domains— molecular virology, immunopathology, endocrine–immune interactions, artificial intelligence–assisted diagnostics, vaccine innovation, and the One Health framework—culminating in a multidisciplinary approach to prevent and control viral diseases in farm animals.*

Chapter 7 – General Conclusions and Recommendations - Comparative Pathobiology of Viral Diseases

7.5 Author's Note

The completion of this book represents a synthesis of years of observation, experimentation, and academic inquiry. It aims to bridge the gap between field pathology and laboratory-based virological research. The author extends appreciation to veterinary scientists and academic institutions dedicated to advancing animal health research and education.

— Prof. Sabaa Hilal Hadi

References

Akhigbe, R. E., Dutta, S., Hamed, M. A., Ajayi, A. F., Sengupta, P., & Ahmad, G. (2022). Viral infections and male infertility: A comprehensive review of oxidative stress. Frontiers in Reproductive Health, 4, 782915.

Alexander, D. J. (2003). Newcastle disease and other avian paramyxoviruses. Rev. Sci. Tech. Off. Int. Epiz., 19(2), 443–462.

Bennett, J. R., Lateef, Z., Fleming, S. B., Mercer, A. A., & Wise, L. M. (2016). Orf virus IL-10 reduces monocyte, dendritic cell, and mast cell recruitment to inflamed skin. Virus Research, 213, 230–237.

Doel, T. R. (2003). FMD vaccines. Virus Research, 91(1), 81–99.

Miller, P. J., Decanini, E. L., & Afonso, C. L. (2010). Newcastle disease: Evolution of genotypes and related diagnostic challenges. Infection, Genetics and Evolution, 10(1), 26– 35.

Comparative Pathobiology of Viral Diseases – Back Matter

Complete References

SABAA HILAL HADI, (2015). MEASUREMENT OF INFECTIOUS DOSE FOR AFTOSA VIRUS ISOLATED FROM IRAQI SHEEP BY INOCULATED THE CHORIO

– ALLANTOIC MEMBRANE OF THE CHICK EMBRYO, ASIAN ACADEMIC RESEARCH JOURNAL OF MULTIDISCIPLINARY, AARJMD, VOLUME 2, ISSUE 1, (JUNE 2015) ISSN : 2319 – 2801.

Doel, T. R. (2003). FMD vaccines. Virus Research, 91(1), 81–99.

Knight-Jones, T. J. D., & Rushton, J. (2013). The economic impacts of foot and mouth disease – What are they, how big are they and where do they occur? Preventive Veterinary Medicine, 112(3–4), 161–173.

Paton, D. J., Valarcher, J. F., Bergmann, I., Matlho, O. G., Zakharov, V. M., Palma, E. L.,& Thomson, G. R. (2009). Selection of foot and mouth disease vaccine strains: A review. Vaccine, 27(4), 32–38.

Rweyemamu, M. M., Roeder, P. L., Mackay, D. K. J., Sumption, K. J., Brownlie, J., Leforban, Y., ... & Valarcher, J. F. (2008). Epidemiological patterns of foot-and-mouth disease worldwide. Transboundary and Emerging Diseases, 55(1), 57–72.

Sumption, K., Rweyemamu, M., & Wint, W. (2008). Incidence and distribution of foot-and-mouth disease in Asia, Africa, and South America. Transboundary and Emerging Diseases, 55(1), 5–13.

Thomson, G. R., Vosloo, W., & Bastos, A. D. S. (2003). Foot and mouth disease in wildlife.Virus Research, 91(1), 145–161.

Sabaa Hilal, Al-Mansory, A. K., & Al-Zobaidy, A. O. (2014). Histological changes in mice (Balb/c) induced by Newcastle Virus. Euphrates Journal of Agriculture Science, 6(Special Issue), 573–584.

Alexander, D. J. (2003). Newcastle disease and other avian paramyxoviruses. Rev. Sci.Tech. Off. Int. Epiz., 19(2), 443–462.

Bhrigu, K., Nagendra, N., Durlav, P., & Sudip, C. (2011). Experimental infection of pigs with group rotavirus and enterotoxigenic Escherichia coli in India: gross, histopathological and immunopathological study. Veterinaria Italiana, 47(2), 117–128.

Debouck, P., & Pensaert, M. (1979). Experimental infection of pigs with Belgian isolates of the porcine rotavirus. Vet. Med. B, 26, 517–526.

Miller, P. J., Decanini, E. L., & Afonso, C. L. (2010). Newcastle disease: Evolution of genotypes and related diagnostic challenges. Infection, Genetics and Evolution, 10(1), 26– 35.

M.A. AL-KHAFAJI, Ghusoon A.A. ALNEAMAH and Sabaa Hilal HADI (2023). Histopathological and Hormonal Assessment of Contagious Ecthyma disease in Rams. International Journal of Applied Sciences and Technology, ISSN: 2717-8234, Volume 5, Issue 3, September 2023, 243–251.

Akhigbe, R. E., Dutta, S., Hamed, M. A., Ajayi, A. F., Sengupta, P., & Ahmad, G. (2022). Viral infections and male infertility: A comprehensive review of oxidative stress. Frontiers in Reproductive Health, 4, 782915.

Bennett, J. R., Lateef, Z., Fleming, S. B., Mercer, A. A., & Wise, L. M. (2016). Orf virus IL-10 reduces monocyte, dendritic cell, and mast cell recruitment to inflamed skin. Virus Research, 213, 230–237.

Li, Y., Wang, X., Bo, K., Wang, X., Tang, B., Yang, B., & Jiang, Y. (2018). PRRSV infection affects testicular function through induction of oxidative stress and apoptosis in boars. Veterinary Microbiology, 219, 93–101.

Nandi, S., De, U. K., & Chowdhury, S. (2011). Current status of contagious ecthyma (orf disease) in goats and sheep: A global perspective. Small Ruminant Research, 96(2), 73– 82.

Beure, K. (2013). Canadian Food Inspection Agency report on foot and mouth disease transmission and control. CFIA Publications.

Reed, L. J., & Muench, H. (1938). A simple method of estimating fifty percent endpoints. American Journal of Hygiene, 27, 493–497.

Thayer, S. G., & Beard, C. W. (2008). Serologic procedures. In A Laboratory Manual for the Identification and Characterization of Avian Pathogens (5th ed., pp. 222–229). American Association of Avian Pathologists.

Acknowledgments

The authors expresses sincere gratitude to academic mentors, colleagues, and research institutions whose indirect contributions helped shape the development of this book. Their commitment to advancing veterinary science and animal health served as a guiding inspiration throughout this project. Appreciation is also extended to reviewers, editors, and readers for their engagement and encouragement. The author remains indebted to the broader scientific community whose foundational work made this synthesis possible.

Comparative Pathobiology of Viral Diseases in Farm Animals: Histopathological and Experimental Insights
offers a comprehensive exploration of three major viral infections affecting farm animals — Foot-and-Mouth Disease Virus (FMDV), Newcastle Disease Virus (NDV), and Orf Virus (ORFV).

Integrating experimental research, histopathological observation, and comparative analysis, this volume provides a detailed examination of how these viruses interact with host tissues, elicit immune responses, and impact both animal health and productivity.

Drawing upon published studies and original experimental data, the book bridges veterinary virology, pathology, and endocrinology, presenting a unified perspective on the

mechanisms of viral pathogenesis across species. Through illustrative figures, tables, and clear academic narrative, it serves as a valuable reference for researchers, veterinarians, and postgraduate students in the fields of microbiology and veterinary sciences.

This work also highlights future directions in comparative viral research, emphasizing the importance of interdisciplinary approaches in controlling and understanding animal viral diseases of global significance.

Sabaa Hilal Hadi

Department of Pathology and Poultry Diseases, Faculty of Veterinary Medicine,
University of Al-Qasim Green, Babylon 51013, Iraq.
E-mail: sabahelal@vet.uoqasim.edu.iq
ORCID: https://orcid.org/0000-0003-2638-9408

FSC
www.fsc.org
MIX
Papier | Fördert gute Waldnutzung
FSC® C083411

Kolibri 360 GmbH
Ferdinand-Jühlke-Straße 7
99095 Erfurt, Deutschland
produktsicherheit@kolibri360.de

Druck:
CPI Druckdienstleistungen GmbH
im Auftrag der
Kolibri 360 GmbH
Ferdinand-Jühlke-Str. 7
99095 Erfurt